LIZ EARLE'S
QUICK GUIDES
Hair Loss

B🌲XTREE

Advice to the Reader

*Before following any advice contained in this book, it is
recommended that you consult your doctor if you suffer from any health
problems or special condition or are in any doubt.*

First published in Great Britain in 1995 by Boxtree Limited,
Broadwall House, 21 Broadwall, London SE1 9PL

10 9 8 7 6 5 4 3 2 1

ISBN: 0 7522 1635 X

Text design by Blackjacks
Cover design by Hammond Hammond

Printed and Bound in Great Britain by Cox & Wyman Ltd.,
Reading, Berkshire

A CIP catalogue entry for this book is available from
the British Library

Contents

ACKNOWLEDGEMENTS

I am grateful to Sheila Lavery for helping to produce this book; also for reference material kindly provided by dermatologist Dr Karen Burke and trichologist Philip Kingsley. I am also grateful to John Firmage MIT, Consultant-in-Charge, The Scalp and Hair Hospital of the Institute of Trichologists. With special thanks to Anthony Maleedy, MIT, consultant trichologist, Dr Hugh Rushton, FIT, consultant trichologist, nutritionist Stephen Terrass, aromatherapist Robert Tisserand and hairdresser Paul Mindle.

Introduction

A great deal of conflicting information has been written and much has been talked about hair. Most experts agree on the basics such as what hair is, how it grows and the factors that affect its growth and appearance, but when it comes to hair loss, opinion divides.

Most experts, but by no means all, agree on how and why hair loss occurs. Unfortunately far fewer agree on how to treat it. The whole area of hair loss, especially in the case of male pattern baldness, is open to constant dispute, change and development. The more orthodox trichologists will opt for drug or surgical treatments and long-established methods only, whereas other practitioners favour newer, more holistic or natural approaches, embracing herbal lotions, nutritional therapy and fundamental changes to lifestyle and diet.

This *Quick Guide* presents the facts on both approaches. It aims to be comprehensive but is by no means exhaustive. When you have read the book, hopefully you will feel more able to choose a treatment that suits you. Whatever the reason for your hair loss, the facts contained in this book will give you the best chance to hold on to a healthy head of hair.

Liz Earle

—1—

A Healthy Head of Hair

The attention that we lavish on our hair on a daily basis is just one indication of how important it is to us. On a very primitive level hair offers protection and warmth, but it also plays a large part in attraction. Beautiful hair has been written and sung about for centuries by everyone from Homer to David Bowie. Hair has also been a status symbol, a sign of power, authority and masculinity; think of a judge's wig and how beards have always indicated maturity and wisdom in men. Hair is also accurately known as a barometer of health; a thick and shiny head of hair is as much a sign of good health and vitality as clear glowing skin, and any ill-health soon registers in the condition of your hair.

Last, but by no means least, hair is a sign of youth. Traditionally, young girls have worn their hair long while mature women wore theirs up or had it cut short to fend off unwanted male attention. In men, too, the first sign of a receding hairline heralds the onset of maturity, an undesirable development in a society where there is so much emphasis on staying young and looking good.

Given all these roles it is small wonder that the loss of hair, either temporarily or permanently, provokes such universal feelings of panic and dread, or that we are prepared to invest so much time, effort and sometimes vast amounts of money to maintain or hopefully regrow it. Consequently, a huge industry of hair growth products and programmes has grown up to feed the desire for a full head of hair. We are offered everything from spray-on hair to micro surgery, and all the lotions and potions in between. This of course is nothing new. It seems that men and women have been losing their hair since time began and for almost all that time there have been 'cures' and disguises for hair loss.

Cures have ranged from Hippocrates' delightful mixture of wine, essence of lilies or roses, oils and acacia juice, to the seventeenth-century practice of rubbing stale urine or white dog droppings on to the scalp. Even chicken manure and electric shock treatment have had a brief, but failed, part to play in scalp stimulation.

Attempts to disguise bald patches also set fashions in hair styles. Think of the classic Roman hairstyle where the hair is brushed forward from the crown and flattened against the scalp. When a balding Roman emperor said it was a new fashion, who was going to argue with him?

Of course, treatments today are much more sophisticated and there is a great deal we can do to maintain, improve and restore thinning hair and balding. As we are learning more about the workings of the human body, how hair grows and why it falls out, we are more aware of what is and is not achievable. Thanks to advances in science, surgical techniques, stress management and nutrition, there is a growing pool of information and help for anyone who needs it. There has also been a growth in understanding among health professionals who are prepared to pay more attention to hair loss than they may have done in the past. A welcome surge of interest in holistic healthcare means that most types of hair loss are seldom seen in isolation. Often it can be a symptom of some underlying health problem and not just a cosmetic change. The message in these cases is that if you boost your health generally, you'll improve the quality of your hair.

Unfortunately, we still have to beware of the quack remedies. Your best defence against squandering your time, money and hope on a useless 'cure' is to be informed. Bear in mind that there are 'treatments' for hair loss as opposed to 'cures'. There is a great deal you can do to improve the condition of your hair, prolong its life and even help it to regrow in some cases, but it pays to be realistic both in your expectations and in the treatments you decide to use.

To understand the problem of hair loss it is important to know a little about the basic structure of hair, how it grows and how that growth cycle changes throughout our lives.

Hair Structure

Hair is made up of **keratin**, a type of fibrous protein which also plays a major role in the formation of nails and the outer layer of our skin. The protein is composed of simpler units called **amino acids**. There is also a proportion of sulphur which contributes to the hard but flexible fibrous appearance. The strands of hair that we can see are actually made up of dead cells and keratin, which is why it never hurts to have your hair cut. But even though they are technically dead, hair strands can still be affected by outside influences such as pollution or the chemicals in hair-styling products.

The root of the hair and part of the shaft is buried beneath the skin in a little pit called the **follicle**. The follicle is the living part of the hair, which is protected and nourished beneath the scalp. The follicle determines the size and shape of each individual hair. At the base of the follicle is the **papilla**, a clump of cells which produce the keratin that forms the hair strands. Each follicle, which develops independently, is surrounded by small blood vessels called capillaries.

Capillaries work in two ways for the follicle. They supply it with nutrients such as vitamins, minerals, water and oxygen and they carry away waste products into the veins or the **lymphatic**

Fig.1

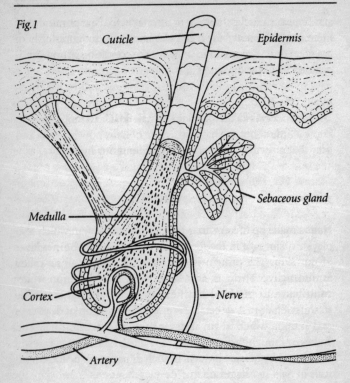

system. The follicle is also linked to a **sebaceous gland**. These are oil-secreting glands which supply a constant flow of sebum (oil) to nourish and moisturise the hair shaft.

The hair shaft itself is divided into three layers: the cuticle, the cortex and the medulla. The cuticle is the outer layer. It is made up of several thinner layers of overlapping cells and is affected by physical and chemical change. The cortex, which is made up of long, thin fibres, forms the bulk of the structure. It contains the main protein-rich part of the hair and the pigments which determine colour. It is also affected by physical and chemical influences which can change it either temporarily or permanently. The medulla is the inner section, a spongy, semi-hollow core. (see Fig.1).

Patterns of Growth and Loss

Hair colour, curliness, thickness and length is hereditary, as is the number of hairs on your head. The average head is host to around 120,000 hairs, although this figure varies depending on colour and race. Blondes have most hairs at around 150,000 and redheads have least with about 90,000, although red hair tends to be coarser so this difference is not usually noticeable.

Our hair pattern is set before birth and we are born with as many hair follicles as we will ever have. Throughout life our hair is constantly growing and renewing itself, at first vigorously, but as we age the rate of growth slows down and so the hair gradually gets thinner. A few follicles die and are not replaced so they will never again produce hair. One thing is certain, we will all lose some hair as we age.

We have different types of hair on different parts of the body and at various stages of our development. As a baby in the womb we are covered with downy hair called **lanugo**, which is usually shed during the ninth month of pregnancy. This is the first of many stages of hair loss. As new-born babies and up until puberty, **vellus hair**, which is fine, short and colourless, covers most of our body. But on our heads, eyebrows and eyelashes we have **terminal hair**, strong, visible, coloured and textured hair. After puberty, hormones trigger the growth of terminal hair in the armpits and pubic area, and on the faces of men.

No matter where it is sited on the body, all hair grows in the same way.

The Life Cycle of Hair

The life cycle of a hair falls into three phases: the anagen, telogen and catagen phases. The **anagen** phase is the period of growth. It lasts for between three and six years. During this time the hair grows continuously at a rate of one to one-and-a-half centimetres a month. The rate of growth can vary, depending on race and inheritance, but generally hair can grow to a length of between 36 centimetres and a metre during the growth phase. Between 85 and 90 percent of hair is in the anagen phase at any time.

Most of the remaining hair is in the resting or **telogen** phase. This period lasts for about three months and during this time the dead hair stays in place until it is pushed out by the new hair. Hair loss occurs in the telogen phase.

The third phase, which is not often mentioned, is called the **catagen** phase. It is a period of regression that lasts for fifteen to twenty days. During this time no new cells are produced. This stage affects only about 1 percent of hair at any time.

We are programmed to have about twenty to twenty-five cycles of growth in our lifetime, depending on our genetic patterning, so how long you keep a full head of hair depends on two basic things: the length of your particular anagen phase (the longer the better) and the quality of the new hair that replaces the hair lost in the telogen phase.

The Influence of Hormones

Although it has never proved desirable as a preventative measure, it is a fact that castration before puberty prevents men going bald. Puberty is a time of increased hormone activity and hormones play an important part in hair growth and hair loss. Generally speaking, oestrogen (a female hormone) has a wonderful effect on hair growth and testosterone (a male hormone) or more accurately **dihydrotestosterone** has the opposite effect. Dihydrotestosterone is a much more potent form of testosterone which occurs when an enzyme called **5 alpha reductase** acts on testosterone. Dihydrotestosterone is usually called androgen and it is an imbalance of this hormone that prevents the hair from growing well and causes hair loss. The reductase enzyme is the inherited factor that influences whether or not you will permanently lose your hair. It can be present in both men and women, but women are offered more protection against genetic hair loss because they have much higher levels of oestrogen than men. The hormone progesterone and its synthetic form progestogen have androgenic properties, so an imbalance can also cause hair loss.

Factors that Affect Hair

The genetic and hormonal influences mentioned above give rise to the most common and probably most distressing form of hair loss called androgenic **alopecia** or male pattern baldness (MPB). MPB can determine the quality, rate of growth and specific patterns of hair loss in both men and women.

Age also affects the quality and quantity of hair. Many men who don't go bald find that their hair thins with age and the loss of pigment in greying hair can result in a less than flattering scatter of dull, coarse hair. Women, too, especially after the menopause, can lose some hair; although they rarely go bald, the hair can get thinner and more brittle. This is a natural consequence of the body slowing down, but it can also be brought on by reduced levels of oestrogen.

Many other factors also affect the appearance, length and quality of our hair. One of the main causes of poor hair growth is badly nourished follicles, caused simply by a lack of nutrients reaching the scalp. Illness, stress, poor nutrition, drugs, hormonal changes and childbirth can all upset the body's metabolism, depriving the cells of the nutrients essential for healthy hair. It is important to remember that it's perfectly normal to lose about 100 hairs a day, but if you notice that you're shedding a lot of hair when you brush or shampoo it and your hair becomes noticeably thinner you should check with your doctor or a **trichologist** (a hair and scalp specialist) to see if this is an abnormal loss. If so, it is important to establish the cause of the loss before you begin to think about treatment.

The Scalp

When talking of hair and hair loss we often forget about the importance of a healthy scalp. Like all skin, the outer layer of the scalp is made up of keratin cells and its natural state is slightly acidic. When the natural balance of the scalp is upset or irritated in any way by harsh shampoos, other chemicals, poor diet or stress, the scalp reacts by producing more keratin, building up dead cells on the scalp which form dandruff (a broad term for many itchy, flaky scalp complaints). Dandruff is a good indicator of stress and stress is one of the main causes of hair loss. It may also be the case that overactive sebaceous glands can contribute to hair loss by eroding the base of the follicle and leaving it more vulnerable to over-vigorous washing, brushing or styling. Most experts agree that in rare cases certain fungal scalp conditions can cause hair loss, by reducing the amount of oxygen getting to the follicles.

—2—
The Causes
of Hair Loss

Trichologists define hair loss in many different ways and by a variety of technical names. On a very simple level there are two basic types of hair loss or alopecia as it is technically termed: physiological and pathological.

Physiological hair loss can be thought of in terms of normal or natural. It occurs as a result of changes within the body. It can be temporary or permanent and tends to be governed by hormonal and ageing factors.

Pathological hair loss is basically due to abnormal factors such as illness, drugs, burns, malnutrition, stress and infection and many other reasons. Details of the more common types are given below.

In order to treat any problem of hair loss correctly it's important to understand the causes. There can, of course, be as many reasons for hair loss as there are people who lose it and a proper diagnosis would involve building up a picture of that person's character, diet and lifestyle to form a complete picture of them and how they react to specific circumstances.

Like every other aspect of life and health, hair loss depends on the individual and while anxiety and stress may cause my hair to fall out, for example, it may have a completely different effect on you. But generally speaking, when there is something wrong in the body, hair is one of the first places to register it. This is because the body has developed a priority system in order to survive and when it is under attack from stress, sickness, drugs or wayward hormones for example, it has to surrender something in order to survive. As hair ranks pretty low in the body's hierarchy of functions, it tends to be sacrificed in favour of the more vital organs.

Listed below are some of the more easily categorised types of hair loss. Most types of hair loss are temporary and usually respond well to treatment. The only types that dermatologists and trichologists consider permanent are certain types of scarring alopecia and androgenic alopecia (male pattern baldness).

Physiological Hair Loss

Physiological hair loss occurs through natural changes in the body. The first loss of this type occurs just after birth when the lanugo hair of a new-born baby is replaced by soft vellus hair. After that the most noticeable physiological changes are the common male pattern baldness, hair loss after pregnancy, during or after the use of the contraceptive pill and at the menopause.

MALE PATTERN BALDNESS

Androgenic alopecia, or male pattern baldness (MPB) as it is commonly known, is probably the most well-known type of baldness and sadly one that causes most anxiety as men and women desperately seek a cure for what has long been considered an incurable condition. About 30 percent of white western males have started to lose some hair by the age of thirty, 40 percent by forty and 50 percent by fifty, so it's not unusual or abnormal, but in a society obsessed with youth and bombarded with multimedia images of square-jawed Grecian gods with full heads of hair, it's difficult to keep the facts in perspective.

It also seems ironic that the society which places so much importance on a full head of hair is the society worst affected. Westerners get a raw deal compared to certain other racial groups. The Japanese, Chinese, American Indians and some African tribes have an amazingly low rate of genetic hair loss.

Since it is impossible to change your race or genetic make-up, hair loss in susceptible men and women is a fact of life. And as we saw in Chapter 1, even those of us who are not affected by genetic baldness do experience some degree of hair loss as a natural part of ageing. It's one of those quirky evolutionary traits that we don't seem able to shake off – the mature chimp sports his receding hairline as a symbol of his maturity and importance, but modern man regards it as less of a status symbol.

Why male pattern baldness occurs

This is a genetic condition, but it doesn't necessarily affect all members of the same family. So, although a cursory glance at the men in your family might give you an indication of how your hair pattern might look in ten or twenty years time, it doesn't necessarily follow that you will definitely be bald because your grandfather or uncles were. You may well have missed out on the gene for baldness. On the other hand, MPB can also affect women, especially in families where there is a high rate of baldness.

As the term suggests, androgenic alopecia is also affected by hormones, specifically the male hormone androgen, which shrinks the hair follicles. Both men and women have male and female hormones. Androgen is responsible for such typically male characteristics such as aggression, coarse and thick facial and body hair and baldness. Obviously men have much more androgen than women, but where there is an imbalance women can also grow facial hair or develop a typically male balding pattern.

It is possible to inherit the baldness gene and keep your hair for many years. Androgenic alopecia doesn't have to strike at twenty-five or thirty, even though many people do go bald at a young age. Often the condition is speeded up by other contributory factors such as stress or illness and the effects of these factors can be slowed down or reversed.

How to recognise MPB

The first signs of hair loss usually occur in puberty. An excessively greasy scalp and hair falling out during washing can be the precursors of male pattern hair loss. Of course, many teenagers

---

THE STAGES OF HAIR LOSS IN MPB

1	A perfect, full head of hair.
2	Slight receding at the front, which can indicate the start of balding in a young man, but will not progress much in an older man.
3	Strong receding hairline at the temples, and thinning hair around the forehead and crown which may not yet be easy to detect.
4	A bald patch starts to appear at the crown and the hair on the forehead area gets even thinner.
5	The thinning and balding forehead and crown area start to join up and a definite horseshoe shape of hair develops around the back and sides.
6	This is a further progression of stage five: the bald patch gradually gets larger and the band of hair around the sides and back gets shorter. There may still be soft, downy (vellus) hairs on the scalp, but these are getting less visible.
7	In extreme cases of hair loss even the horseshoe of hair at the back and sides can dwindle away.

Adapted from the Hamilton Scale

---

have greasy hair and as we've seen in Chapter 1 we all lose some hair every day, but genetic hair loss is different because there is a heavier than normal hair fall and the hair's thickness, length and quality gradually start to change.

This is a very gradual process. The old, thick and visible hair falls out in the telogen phase as always and is replaced with new hair that grows in the anagen phase. But because of the choking effect that androgen has on the follicle, the new hair is slightly thinner,

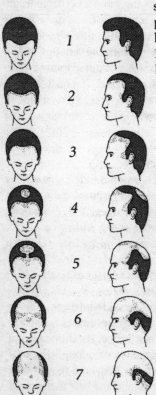

shorter and weaker. As each cycle progresses so each new anagen hair gets less and less visible. Eventually you are left with vellus hairs (like a baby's hair) instead of the terminal hair you started with – sometimes you will have completely dead follicles.

MPB develops in a recognisable pattern, beginning with strong receding at the temples. As 96 percent of boys and 80 percent of girls experience some recession at puberty as a natural result of hormonal activity, you do have to look for a pronounced recession. Next the hair gets thinner around and above the forehead and a bald patch starts to appear at the crown. Gradually the bald patch gets bigger so that only a diminishing horseshoe shape of hair remains around the sides and back of the head. This occurs in what trichologists break down into an eight-stage scale known as the Hamilton Scale, a system of reference devised by dermatologist James Hamilton. You will often see it as a seven-point scale as is shown here (see box), or sometimes even as a five-point scale.

HAIR LOSS AFTER PREGNANCY

The technical term for hair loss after pregnancy is post-partum alopecia. This is perfectly normal and occurs in up to 45 percent of new mothers. But it can be worrying when it occurs in frightening proportions and anxiety about hair loss can make it even worse (stress is probably the most common cause of serious hair loss). If you find you are losing an alarming amount of hair shortly after giving birth try not to worry about it; remind yourself that it is normal and that it will grow back. If it really bothers you, you could ask your doctor to refer you to a trichologist. Specialist treatment can sometimes slow down the hair loss and speed up regrowth.

Why we lose hair after pregnancy

Think back to how the balance of hormones differentiates male from female. Androgen, as we've seen, is responsible for certain male characteristics. Oestrogen, on the other hand, is a quieter hormone that enables women to be softer and more placid, characteristics that are important during pregnancy. It is also one that is needed for an abundance of healthy hair.

During pregnancy a woman produces more oestrogen, which alters the balance of the body, making sure that she leads a quieter life for the benefit of her baby. It also tends to interfere with the hair's growth cycle so that even though she produces new hairs, she doesn't always lose the old ones, hence the abundance of glossy healthy hair that makes pregnant women look so blooming. Soon after pregnancy, however, the body and its wayward hormones start to go back to normal and the hair that should have been shed during pregnancy falls out with a vengeance.

How to recognise post-partum alopecia

The hair loss usually begins between two and seven months after the birth. It occurs in a similar way to male pattern baldness: balding at the hairline, receding at the temples and generally thinning over the whole scalp area. Women who breastfeed will notice that their loss occurs when they stop or cut down on their baby's feeds.

HAIR LOSS AND THE PILL

Some women notice that they lose hair as a side-effect of taking the contraceptive pill; others whose hair is abundantly healthy while taking the pill notice a worrying loss of hair when they stop taking it. The pill introduces synthetic hormones to the body which knock the body's own hormones out of balance, so hair growth can often be affected in one of two ways. The first occurs in women who lose hair while they're on the pill. This is not so common in these days of low-progestogen pills, but it can still occur. The pill can be a combination of oestrogen and progestogen (a synthetic form of progesterone) or progestogen only. As we saw in Chapter 1, progestogen causes hair loss because of its androgenic characteristics. The solution is to switch to a low-progestogen pill or come off the pill altogether.

The second form of hair loss happens in women who have been receiving high levels of oestrogen from their contraceptive pill. It tends to occur about three months after coming off the pill, in a similar way to post-partum hair loss. Once off the pill the body's oestrogen levels settle down and quite a lot of hair can be lost. It will take a few months to return to normal.

MENOPAUSAL HAIR LOSS

Again, it comes down to hormones. It seems that hair loss, which has traditionally been considered a male problem, is one that women have to battle with at every stage of their life. During the menopause, oestrogen production gradually slows down until it stops altogether. The menopause upsets the body's hormonal balance so that androgen becomes more dominant and oestrogen less so. Consequently, some women notice that the hair on their heads gets thinner, while the vellus hair on the chin and upper lip can get coarser and darker. If the menopause occurs quickly the hair loss will also be quick, so it's more noticeable and consequently more stressful; a slower menopause will result in a more gradual, diffuse loss where the hair thins out over a long period of time.

The pattern of hair loss is similar to that of male pattern baldness and, like male pattern baldness, stress makes the problem worse. Unfortunately, the menopause is a time of tremendous stress for many women. This change of life can and should be a time of joy, independence and liberation, but too often it is seen as the end of youth, attractiveness and fulfilment. Not surprisingly many women feel anxious and depressed and hair loss can be symptomatic of both.

Menopausal hair loss is not necessarily permanent. As the hormones gradually stabilise some of the hair may grow back, but it's unlikely to return to its pre-menopausal abundance.

Pathological Hair Loss

The types of pathological hair loss can be further divided into three basic groups: cicatrical alopecia, telogen effluvium and anagen defluvium. These all have very technical names but the scientific theory is quite straightforward.

CICATRICAL ALOPECIA

This unpronounceable name simply means hair loss caused by scarring. This means the hair follicles are damaged and will never be able to produce hair. It can be due to defects that occurred during development in the womb or as a result of disease or trauma such as burns to the scalp.

TELOGEN EFFLUVIUM

This type of hair loss has several causes. It occurs when the growth (anagen) phase ends abruptly so that the hair quickly passes through the resting (catagen) and falling (telogen) phases. In short, it is lost before its time. The hair loss is rarely permanent and usually affects less than 50 percent of the hairs at any one time, so it doesn't normally lead to baldness. But in severe cases of chronic hair loss (where the hair loss occurs over a long period of time) your genetic allowance of growth cycles may be used up so that the hair remains permanently thin.

Stress is the main cause of telogen effluvium. The hair loss usually takes place about three months after the event or factor that caused it, which is why it is often difficult to pinpoint the exact cause.

Stress is recognised by all dermatologists, trichologists and alternative practitioners as a major contributory factor in hair loss. It is a threat to mental and physical health and one to which none of us is immune. Under stress the body's defence system roars into action and hair is often the first casualty. Stress can severely affect how the body functions. It interferes with the normal metabolic process, and deprives the hair follicles of the nutrients they need to grow. This happens through a process called **vasoconstriction** which literally means that the blood vessels carrying nutrients around the body tighten so that nutrients can't flow through to the hair follicle which eventually starves.

Traction alopecia is a form of telogen effluvium and the most common type of hair loss in black people. It is literally hair that is pulled out by the root and in severe cases this can result in permanent hair loss. Traction alopecia occurs when hair is continually styled in a tight bun, ponytails or braids or simply brushed too hard. Children are particularly susceptible because their hair is more fragile than that of adults and they are more likely to have their hair pulled back tight and tied in rubber bands, ribbons and hair slides.

The pattern of hair loss in traction alopecia is a receding frontal hairline. It can also be seen in the partings of women who habitually part their hair in the middle and scrape it into a bun at the back. Banded alopecia is a variation on traction alopecia common in black girls who have their hair straightened or plaited tightly in rows. The constant tension on the hair causes it to break off all round the edge of the scalp. It can also be pulled out along a parting.

ANAGEN DEFLUVIUM

In anagen defluvium hair loss occurs because the hair shafts become thin and break. Unlike telogen effluvium, this type of hair loss usually begins between a few days and a few weeks after the causative event or factor and can be much more severe, affecting up to 90 percent of the hairs at any one time. The condition is not usually permanent if it is treated. It affects men and women of all races.

Alopecia areata is the most common form of this type of hair loss. This is the name given to a type of hair loss that causes round patches of hair loss on the scalp, or in the beard or eyebrows, which get bigger as the disease develops.

It can be either acute or chronic and is usually the result of physical or mental trauma such as a major shock, surgery, severe dieting and certain types of drugs. Anticoagulants (used to treat and prevent abnormal blood clotting); amphetamines (stimulants) and anticonvulsants (used in the treatment of epilepsy and other types of seizure) can all cause patches of hair loss. Poor nutrition and illnesses that affect the endocrine system (such as thyroid problems, diabetes and certain cancers) are a common cause. People with Down's syndrome are particularly vulnerable to alopecia areata and there is a strong link between the disease and vitiligo.

Nutrition is also a factor. What you take into your body can affect what happens to your hair and it's not so much a case of you are what you eat as you are what you absorb. For more information on the importance of diet turn to Chapter 5. Apart from nutritional deficiencies, vitamin poisoning such as excessive amounts of vitamin A can also cause this type of hair loss.

Hair Breakage

Hair that breaks off at the scalp can result in a thin, patchy look, but it is not hair loss in the strict sense and is often referred to as hair fall. It usually occurs as a result of damage to the hair and can be so extensive as to look like balding. The hair becomes dry and brittle, stripped of its oily protection and deprived of moisture. This results in the fibres within the hair shaft splitting and breaking.

There are various causes of excessive dry and fragile hair, from too little **sebum** to central heating and sunbathing. But hair usually breaks as a result of mistreatment. Perming, bleaching, overzealous washing and styling with heated products can all cause dull, dry and brittle hair. Severely damaged hair needs intensive treatment such as that mentioned in Chapter 3, but in most cases just follow the rules in Chapter 5 to keep hold of your hair.

Compulsive hair pulling (known as trichotillomania) can also result in bald patches. But this condition, which can be a symptom of neglect, is more psychological than physical. Hair care is important, but the first step is to find out why someone feels the need to mutilate themselves in this way.

Other Causes and the Latest Research

The most common and well-established causes of hair loss have been discussed above, but there are of course many more.

Severe illness and radical medical treatment such as chemotherapy can cause temporary hair loss, as can many types of drugs. Fungal infections, such as dermatitis of the scalp and ringworm can also cause hair loss although these are now rare. Chemicals and diseases such as lupus can all have an effect because they affect the body's metabolism. We can even be born with damaged follicles.

Advances in medicine continue to establish more and more links and current British research indicates that there may be a link between male pattern baldness and heart disease in men and between hair loss and ovarian disorders and infertility in women.

Hairline International operate a telephone helpline dedicated to alopecia (see Useful Addresses).

Myths About Baldness

Wearing a cap will make you go bald. This fallacy probably arises from the fact that many bald men wear caps to cover their bald patches and keep their heads warm. It is not very healthy to keep your scalp covered at all times as your skin needs to breathe, but a cap won't make your hair fall out unless it is so tight as to cause traction alopecia.

Shaving your head will prevent baldness. Another fallacy that probably arises from the idea that shaving your hair makes it grow back thicker. It doesn't. Your hair thickness and density of coverage are determined by your genes, a quick flick with a razor won't change that. However, keeping your hair short and layered can make it look thicker.

Greasy hair will go bald. For a long time it was thought that greasy hair, caused by an excess of sebum, was the precursor to hair loss. In fact, male pattern baldness used to be called seborrhoeic alopecia. But the official stance is that even though greasy hair and male pattern hair loss are both androgen related, they are quite separate conditions and one doesn't necessarily lead to the other. However, certain conditions such as seborrhoeic eczema can cause hair loss in rare cases.

Bald men are more virile. Many balding men have quite heavy body hair due to the activity of high levels of male hormones. This 'macho man' image coupled with the idea of surging testosterone has given rise to the idea of super-virile baldies. Sorry boys, the hormone activity is far more likely to make you aggressive and stressed out than heighten your manly vigour.

Women don't go bald. Yes they do, but often in a different way and the reason for it is often harder to detect. Almost 60 percent of women suffer hair loss at some time in their lives and we all lose hair as we get older. Women can develop male pattern baldness in the same stages as men but very often it is what is known as **diffuse alopecia**, ie general thinning all over the scalp. Women in the 1990s are as susceptible to stress as men are and are just as likely to have an unhealthy lifestyle. Women normally have eight parts of oestrogen (for hair) to one part androgen (for hair loss), but this ratio can fluctuate at various stages of life and hair loss can result.

Baldness is inherited from your mother. You can inherit the baldness gene from either side of your family, although it may be more likely to come from your mother's family. But baldness is a variable trait. Your brother may go bald while you retain a full head of hair well into old age.

— 3 —

Can Hair Loss Be Cured?

Most types of acute hair loss can be cured and some hair simply grows back in its own time, without any help. But there is no miracle cure for hair loss, and many of the treatments that do work don't work in all cases. The first step in preventing hair loss and encouraging new growth is to find out the cause of your problem and for this you need to get professional advice and treatment. You could go to your GP or usual health practitioner and many people do, but it may be best to go to a hair specialist, known as a trichologist.

How to Find a Trichologist

Trichology is the scientific study and treatment of hair and a trichologist is a trained practitioner who specialises in diagnosing and treating hair disorders. He or she is not a hairdresser. There are many people who call themselves trichologists or hair specialists and legally anyone can set up in business as a trichologist so it pays to be cautious. Always look for a registered trichologist who is a member of the Institute of Trichologists. The Institute was founded in 1902 and is the governing body that lays down the code of conduct and practice which all its members must follow. A trichologist who is a member of the Institute will have completed a minimum of three years study involving clinical training and practice and will have the letters

AIT, MIT or FIT after their name, indicating that they are either an Associate Member, Member or Fellow of the Institute.

Trichologists work privately and fees vary according to the practitioner and treatment, but you can expect to pay a minimum of £25 for a consultation and at least £13 for an hour's treatment. You will also have to pay for any specialist products you need to use at home. The Institute forbids registered trichologists from advertising so there's no point in looking in the small ads. To find a trichologist in your area you will need to contact the Secretary at the Institute of Trichologists in London (see Useful Addresses).

What a Trichologist Can Do For You

All the experts agree that your chances of stopping or even reversing hair loss can be greatly improved if you get treatment as soon as possible.

Trichologists report that an increased number of people are taking advantage of their specialist skills to find solutions to a whole range of hair problems. Trichologists don't believe this increase is due to more people having hair and scalp problems, rather they put it down to the fact that people are more aware; fewer are prepared to put up with poor quality hair because they know there are treatments available that do work. Even people whose hair is in excellent condition visit trichologists occasionally to be pampered or to pre-empt hairloss problems by improving the health of their hair.

If you have a problem with hair loss, it might be worth making an appointment with a trichologist who may be able to see a side to your problems that you have missed. You might think your hair loss is due to a bad perm but that may be only an indirect cause, the real problem could be something altogether different. Modern hair care is, and indeed has to be,

holistic – it must take into consideration all aspects of your life from birth until the present, not just what you have put on your head in the last six months. An accurate diagnosis is the beginning and most vital step in treating the problem.

What Happens When You Visit a Trichologist?

CONSULTATION

A first visit starts with a consultation. The therapist will talk to you to find out what has happened in your life recently, if you've been ill, are on medication, have had a baby, had an accident, a shock or a stressful experience, or if there is a history of baldness in your family. Good therapists will pick up on your levels of anxiety and reassure you about your chances of successful treatment. If, for example in the case of advanced male pattern baldness, they feel there is little apart from radical surgery that will improve the look of your hair, they will encourage you to accept your condition. In fact acceptance is important even if you do go on to receive further treatment. If you accept that the worst that can happen is that you will still be bald at the end of it then you are unlikely to be disappointed by any improvements, however small or slow they may be. Improving, regrowing or restoring hair is a slow and sometimes painful process, you have to be patient and realistic.

EXAMINATION

The examination is actually part of the consultation but it's easier to treat it as the second step. The trichologist will examine your hair and scalp with a magnifying glass or under a microscope if necessary. About 98 percent of the time they can tell what is wrong with the hair just by looking at it, but occasionally the client may need to have a blood test or see their GP. In the case of male pattern baldness, this condition will follow a certain pattern as indicated by the Hamilton Scale mentioned in Chapter 2. The trichologist will determine where you register on the scale before discussing your treatment options and deciding on a course of treatment.

Apart from male pattern baldness the other major difference is whether the hair fall is due to loss or breakage. The difference is usually determined by the elasticity of the hair. Hair that breaks has poor elasticity because the quality of the outer cellular structure of the hair shafts has deteriorated to become so dry and brittle that it can literally break off at the scalp. Incorrect combing or brushing, harsh styling products or overprocessing with perms and colourants can all contribute to or worsen already brittle hair. To the untrained eye hair fall caused by hair breaking off at the scalp can easily be mistaken for true alopecia (hair loss from the follicle), but to an expert armed with magnifying equipment it's easier to detect. One difference is that hair strands lost through alopecia will usually have a little white fleshy bulb that broken hairs won't have.

In rare cases the hair loss may be due to a fungal infection on the scalp. If the problem is neither MPB nor hair breakage it is likely to be one of the many forms of temporary alopecia detailed in Chapter 2. The consultation which includes taking details about your health, diet and lifestyle should reveal the specific condition.

TREATMENT

Treatment can depend as much on the individual as on the type of hair loss they are experiencing. But most centres tend to use a selection of treatments to nourish the hair, improve its condition and the condition of the scalp and to stimulate regrowth. Listed below are the basic treatments offered by a trichologist. Sometimes a therapist will have a preference for a specific treatment not mentioned here. You may also find that some trichologists have developed their own products and hair-care systems that are exclusive to their own clinic.

Stimulating the blood circulation is important for all types of hair loss because a healthy blood flow improves the chances of nutrients getting to the hair follicles. Trichologists do this either with actino or ray therapy (treatment with light) or with a vibro massager. Actino therapy can involve either ultraviolet light, radiant heat or infra-red light depending on the type and severity of the condition. Basically, infra-red waves are long waves of light which are more soothing and calming than stimulating; radiant heat uses shorter waves of light that are slightly stronger; and ultraviolet light uses very short rays that are highly penetrating and very stimulating. Even though ultraviolet treatment uses very strong rays there is virtually no heat, which makes it comfortable but very dangerous: you could sit under a UV light for hours without feeling any burning sensation yet emerge with a completely scorched and blistered scalp. To an expert it is a useful tool for boosting blood flow to the scalp without damaging the scalp or the hair, but in the hands of an amateur it can be a dangerous weapon. The effect and feeling of actino or ray therapy is similar to the blood rush that you feel when you hang your head upside down.

Similar effects can be achieved with a vibro massager, a hand-held electrical massager that can also be beneficial in the hands of an expert. If you want to massage your scalp at home see the section on massage in Chapter 5.

Alopecia areata – sometimes a trichologist will treat patches of baldness such as those in alopecia areata with a combination of massage and a **vasodilation** lotion such as methylnicotinate. This process boosts circulation and encourages a quicker regrowth. When the hair starts to grow back the tip is colourless so it's difficult to see the new hair, but the colour returns within a very short time. Some pigment should start to show after two weeks, so as the hair grows it will gradually return to its original colour.

Fungal infections such as dermatitis or severe dandruff can cause hair loss but these conditions are not very common in these days of scrupulous hygiene. Most people keep their dandruff under control by over-the-counter coal tar preparations or anti-dandruff shampoos which clear away the dead cells on the surface of the scalp. Only in rare cases does the infection become a threat to the health of your hair. Then a trichologist would use an antiseptic, which has an anti-mitotic effect (it slows down the division of cells that cause the dandruff rather than just clearing them away).

Male pattern baldness and hair thinning in women is also treated with relative success. Trichologists recognise how distressing this type of hair loss can be, especially to women. It can cause loss of confidence and self-esteem. In the past there was relatively little anyone could do, but recent treatments involving the topical application of oestrogen creams can arrest the problem and improve regrowth for about 30 percent of women and 20 percent of men.

Post-partum hair loss usually stops as suddenly as it started and follows the recognised regrowth pattern, so there is usually no need for treatment. However, in very rare cases where the hair fall is exceptionally heavy or it continues beyond the eighth month after giving birth, professional treatment can be successful. Such cases usually occur because of hormonal imbalance, perhaps these women had a high androgen level to start with which was triggered by the pregnancy. Treatment would be similar to that given for male pattern baldness.

Hair loss due to breakage can be caused by ill-health or biological changes that aren't immediately apparent and finding the true cause would determine the type of treatment. But most cases are due to neglect or harsh treatment – they are self-inflicted and quite easy to reverse with a little tender loving care. Blow drying, perming, swimming and sunbathing all strip the hair of its natural oils leaving it dull, dry and vulnerable to further damage. If your hair is severely damaged and broken, a trichologist would usually recommend you have your hair trimmed, giving you an intensive conditioning treatment to smooth down the surface of the hair shaft so that it is immediately more manageable and less susceptible to future damage. This may be followed by dietary and general advice on how to care for your hair (see Chapter 5).

Scarring alopecia – unfortunately, this condition is unlikely to benefit from anything apart from surgery. It is important to consult a trichologist to start with; he or she will refer you to a reputable surgeon if you want to consider this option.

Dietary advice – trichologists give specific nutritional advice to clients and some clinics, such as the Trichological Centre in Manchester (see Useful Addresses) will send free information to anyone who requests it on feeding your hair and scalp. For more advice on the benefits of healthy eating turn to Chapter 5.

Alternative Treatments

Many alternative practitioners have had significant success with hair loss problems. If you want to avoid drug treatments or are more interested in boosting your general health and well-being, holistic treatment from an alternative or complementary practitioner could give your hair the kick-start it needs.

If you can't decide whether you want aromatherapy, homoeopathy, herbalism, acupuncture or nutritional medicine or any of the many other forms of treatment, think in terms of which treatment you feel most comfortable with as opposed to which treatment works best for hair loss. This is because there is no one treatment that works best for hair loss, just one that works best for you.

Holistic medicine is not like orthodox medicine, you don't match the symptoms with the treatment, because the symptoms are only part of the picture. You, and all aspects of your mental, physical and emotional health, are the whole picture. If the treatment works for you it will work for your hair. To find out more about holistic health, contact the Institute for Complementary Medicine or the British Complementary Medicine Association (see Useful Addresses).

If none of the above treatments works to your satisfaction trichologists can discuss transplantation and other surgical options with you. Their willingness to refer you to a surgeon will depend on a number of factors including whether they believe you are a suitable candidate for surgery; for example, do you have enough hair to transplant and are your expectations realistic? If you want to pursue any of the surgical options detailed in Chapter 4 always make sure you go to a recommended surgeon – if you don't the results can be disastrous.

When to See a Professional

If your hair has lost elasticity. Healthy hair should stretch to between 25 and 35 percent of its length before it breaks. To test this take a hair from your head and stretch it between two fingers along the length of a ruler. Measure how much it stretched before it broke – if it is less than 25 percent you've got dry hair that needs treating.

If you are losing more than 100 hairs a day. As mentioned already some hair loss is normal and healthy, but heavy hair fall is not. You are not expected to count your hairs one by one, but if it seems that you are losing more than about 100 hairs a day and you notice your hair getting thinner then you are experiencing hair loss. If you want to stop the hair loss you are advised to get professional help.

If you've tried everything available to you without success. You can make changes to your diet, try over-the-counter products, massage or alternative treatments and you may have some success, but you do need to recognise when self-help measures are not working.

Any time there is a sudden or abnormal change to the hair. Sudden or exceptionally heavy hair loss is not normal. It can be the result of physical or psychological trauma and needs to be investigated for the sake of your health if not your hair.

If you are worried. This is probably the most important reason of all. There is no need to sit at home worrying about the state of your hair when there is help available. Whatever the problem, worrying will only make it worse. No matter how small or large your problem is, something can be done to make you feel better about it.

4

Hair Loss Treatments for Male Pattern Baldness

In the case of male pattern baldness where the hair loss is considered permanent, there are genuine forms of treatments competing for attention in an absolute minefield of quack remedies that at best offer nothing but false hope and at worst can cause lasting damage. So how do you know which are genuine? Quite simply you have two choices; you can play safe and follow the orthodox line of thinking or you can examine all the evidence for what's available from both conventional and alternative practitioners and decide what seems the best option for you.

If you decide to stick with the orthodox view you have a choice of drug treatment or surgery. Although trichologists believe that an improvement in stress levels, nutrition or lifestyle can reverse hair loss in some cases, they do not believe such improvement can prevent hair loss or cause hair to grow back if you've been genetically programmed to lose it. Some alternative hair growers think differently. This chapter discusses both options: the orthodox and the alternative. Of course, it is impossible to cover every alternative treatment on offer, but this selection includes some of the more feasible treatments which have clinical trials to back up their claims.

Drug Treatment

Of the drug treatments available, the one that has been shown to be the most effective is minoxidil, which is marketed as a lotion called Regaine. Minoxidil is a bit of a mystery because unlike its predecessors – oestrogen and progesterone treatments – it is not a hormone or even a hormone-based drug. Even trichologists don't know how or why it works but it does have some success.

Minoxidil was originally prescribed as an oral treatment for high blood pressure before it was found to promote hair growth in parts of the body that didn't normally sport a vigorous crop, such as the forehead, cheeks and arms. So what prompted a shriek of horror in hundreds of people with high blood pressure brought a cry of delight from a whole bevy of balding men and women.

A subsequent clinical trial in America confirmed the good news and minoxidil (Regaine) is available on prescription in this country. But although minoxidil can help some people it is not a wonder drug so, before you rush off to your GP, acquaint yourself with these basic facts about minoxidil.

* Estimates vary but it has a success rate of between 5 and 20 percent.

* It is better at arresting hair loss than treating it, so it's more effective for younger men who have started to go bald in the last five years.

* It does not appear to work on a receding hairline.

* It works best on small bald patches.

* You have to apply it twice a day for four months to notice any improvement.

* You have to continue to apply it twice a day to maintain the improvement.

* If you stop applying minoxidil you will go back to your original level of baldness in three to six weeks.

* It is available only on prescription. Products advertised in newspapers and magazines which claim to contain minoxidil are either making false claims or are illegal.

* It is a drug and all drugs have side-effects. On a day-to-day level it can cause hypersensitivity to sunlight in susceptible individuals and sometimes itching of the scalp, but the long-term effects of using it are not yet known.

OTHER DRUG-BASED TREATMENTS

Oestrogen. Topical application of synthetic oestrogen is not as popular as it used to be. In the early days of treating hair loss, men were sometimes fed oestrogen, but this was soon dropped when some men started to develop female sex characteristics. One way round the problem was to apply oestrogen creams or lotions to the balding areas of the scalp instead. Oestrogen creams are quite a popular form of treatment in trichological clinics, but are not popular with everyone. Like minoxidil, oestrogen creams have to be applied to the scalp every day and used indefinitely. They have a similar success rate to minoxidil.

Anti-androgens. Experiments are being carried out on anti-androgens – drugs which inhibit the production of testosterone. Anti-androgens are not widely available and need to be handled with care as there can be considerable side-effects. According to consultant trichologist Dr Hugh Rushton, anti-androgens are the only drugs that can actually reverse hair loss. Clinical trials have shown that, although it doesn't reverse hair loss in men, it can stop further loss in 90 percent of cases. For obvious reasons men cannot take anti-androgens internally, but they can have it applied topically by a suitably qualified professional (Dr Rushton uses this treatment – see Useful Addresses – but doesn't know of anyone else who does). Women can take the drug internally, and have a much better success rate. In clinical trials between 30 and 40 percent of women actually grew their hair back.

Finasteride. The latest development on the drug scene is with a drug called finasteride, marketed as Proscar. Proscar has long been regarded as a safe, accepted prescription treatment for men with benign prostatic hyperplasia (enlarged prostate), a condition which tends to affect older men. Recent research claims that Proscar can encourage hair growth. Prostates get enlarged because of the action of dihydrotestosterone, the same hormone that affects hair loss. Proscar knocks out the enzyme 5 alpha reductase, which converts testosterone into dihydrotestosterone, so theoretically it should also inhibit balding. But Proscar is not licensed as a treatment for hair loss and is generally considered unsuitable for younger sexually active men. There are mixed views on whether Proscar actually works as a treatment for hair loss, and it can damage the development of a foetus in the womb, if a woman has conceived with sperm carrying the drug. Proscar has been found in male sperm and it can stay in a man's body for up to eight weeks after he has stopped taking the drug.

Dianette. Women who are losing hair through androgenic hair loss may benefit from the contraceptive pill Dianette. It works by preventing androgen-dependent problems from expressing themselves. It is not an incredibly successful treatment but is more effective when backed up by extra cyproterone acetate (a steroid). All the usual side-effects of taking the contraceptive pill apply to taking Dianette.

Surgical Options

When all other methods fail surgery may be the only way to halt the visible signs of hair loss. In the case of male pattern baldness, trichologists regard hair transplants as the only lasting way to correct hair loss. But it's important to remember that surgery is a serious and expensive business, not something to be entered into lightly or without proper consultation.

Not everyone is suitable for transplants. There are certain points that a trichologist would consider before considering someone for surgery.

* The quantity of hair. It's vital to have enough hair at the back and sides of the head to allow the surgeon to remove sections of it and transplant it to the balding areas of the scalp, because hair transplant simply means redistributing what hair you have – it does not introduce new hair.

* Age and attitude. The age and mental attitude of the patient is also important. A twenty-year-old man with advanced hair loss may be destined to lose even more hair from all over his scalp in which case hair transplantation would be a waste of time, money and may end up as an unsightly mess. When transplanted hair is lost it leaves ugly scars so that the unfortunate person is not only poorer and bald, but scarred as well.

* Expectations. As we get older our expectations change. A twenty-year-old may expect miraculous results from

transplantation and be disappointed with what is achievable, whereas a forty-five-year-old may have more realistic expectations. Trichologists are always wary of people who expect miracles.

WHAT'S ON OFFER?

There are several choices of surgical treatment and those choices depend very much on the extent and the site of the hair loss. Sometimes more than one type of treatment is used and several sessions of treatment are often required before you can achieve a finished look.

Transplant techniques are becoming increasingly sophisticated and success rates are high, but so is the cost and sometimes the pain factor. You can expect to pay up to £5,000 for hair surgery and there is a certain amount of discomfort involved.

However, if the candidate is suitable, most hair transplants do work. During transplant surgery the hair complete with the living follicle and surrounding tissue is removed from a growing site, such as the back and sides of the head, and transplanted to a balding site. There it acts as if it were still in its original site. The result of skilled surgery is usually quite a convincing head of hair. The hair in the site from which the grafts were removed will be thinner as no new hair will grow there, but the overall look is usually quite natural.

Punch grafting

This is the most common type of grafting. It involves taking small (4mm) plugs of scalp containing between fifteen and twenty hairs, follicles and surrounding tissue from the back of the scalp where the hair is usually more plentiful and transplanting it into smaller holes in the balding areas of the scalp. Depending on the size of the bald patch it can take up to three transplantation sessions of four or five hours surgery each time to produce a convincing growth pattern over the bald area. Each operation must be at least three months apart. About fifty to sixty plugs are transplanted in each session which means that a total of about 3,500 hairs could be relocated to produce a thinner but more even coverage.

Micrografting and minigrafting

Both techniques are very convincing for receding at the hairline. They are performed in the same way as punch grafting, but use much smaller sections of hair. Minigrafts use plugs of four to seven hairs and micrografts use minuscule plugs of just two or three hairs. These tiny grafts are implanted with tweezers into slits rather than holes. The result is a much more natural look along the hair line, avoiding the artificial look created by punch grafting.

Scalp reduction

This technique is used on the typical Friar Tuck bald spot at the crown. It involves cutting away a central section of the bald patch and pulling together the sides so that the total bald area is significantly reduced. As with punch grafting, it often takes more than one operation. A very bald man may need several scalp reductions, where the scalp is stretched little by little, so that the bald area becomes small enough to be transplanted with punch grafts. If you are cringing at the very thought of it, it's hardly surprising; scalp reduction is a severe and very painful way to get rid of your bald spot.

Flap grafting

If the thought of scalp reduction set your teeth on edge, then you might be advised to skip this section on flap grafting. As the name suggests a flap graft involves a flap of scalp being grafted from one area to another, namely from a hair-growing area to a bald patch in a similar way to skin grafting. This is a drastic operation and not a very popular one as it doesn't give a very natural finish at the hairline in the way that micrografting does and also because the hairs on the flap grow in a different direction from the rest of the hair around it, giving the effect of a wig.

Soft tissue expansion

One of the latest developments in scalp surgery is soft tissue expansion. Although it doesn't sound very appealing, it is a useful technique especially in patients who have lost their hair through scarring or burns. As the name suggests the scalp is stretched by means of silicon bags which are inserted under the hairy areas of the scalp and gradually filled with salt water over a period of between two and four months. The areas of scalp still growing hair slowly expand until the bags are removed. The bald patch is then cut out and replaced with a flap of hair from the stretched area.

A WORD OF WARNING

The success of a transplant rests in the hands of the surgeon. These intricate operations require an incredible amount of time and skill. It is important that the transplant plug is angled and transplanted correctly so that the hair looks like it is growing naturally. When transplants fail, it is either because the sections that were transplanted were destined to be lost anyway or, more likely, because the operation was performed incorrectly. So if you are considering a transplant it is essential to see a fully qualified and experienced transplant surgeon. Go to someone who has been recommended by a trichologist or your GP.

AFTER SURGERY

Transplants need a short settling-in period. After surgery the repopulated areas of the scalp will be covered with a crusty scab for a few days. Then, after two–four weeks, the donor hairs fall out and new hairs grow over the next couple of months. Tests have shown that the rate of regrowth can be speeded up if minoxidil is applied to the scalp after surgery.

It's important to take care of yourself after surgery. Any operation, no matter how small, is an assault on the body and there is so much that complementary treatments can offer to ease the trauma. Why not enjoy a relaxing aromatherapy massage once a week while you're waiting for your new hair to grow or see a homoeopath who can prescribe a post-operative remedy to get your body back in balance. Remember, also, to relax and eat well. Stress and poor nutrition are your hair's enemies and no operation, no matter how sophisticated, will be a success if you don't look after your body's basic requirements.

Weaving

Weaving is a cosmetic technique as opposed to a surgical one. It is not as popular as it was about ten years ago and is not recommended by reputable trichologists for reasons that will become apparent. Sections of your own hair are interwoven with synthetic strands to make the hair look thicker. The advantages are that it is immediately effective, and because the weave is much more permanent than a hairpiece would be, you can carry on swimming, sleeping or exercising as normal. But there are disadvantages which deserve much more consideration. First of all the weave covers the scalp so it is very difficult to get to the scalp underneath. Consequently, the scalp doesn't get cleaned or massaged which can often lead to a heavy build-up of severe dermatitis, which is unhygienic and unhealthy. Also, because the weave is attached to real hair it gradually moves away from the scalp as the hair grows and has to be repositioned several times a year which is an inconvenient and expensive process. Ultimately it may also be a self-defeating one as constant pulling and stretching the hair can cause traction alopecia, so you could lose even more hair than you started out with.

The Alternative Approach

Exploring the alternatives is where the difficulties start. If you decide to try an alternative treatment the key word is caution. The whole area of hair loss treatment is ripe for exploitation. People who are desperate to keep their hair are often vulnerable and easy prey to unscrupulous sales people, and although there are many claims there is very little evidence. Because of the wealth of conflicting claims and information it's important to be informed when deciding to follow an alternative approach. You need to know what type of hair loss you have and what you can realistically expect to achieve. Some products which claim to cure hair loss probably can help with certain types of temporary hair loss but a question mark still hangs over whether they can reverse permanent loss such as that caused by male pattern baldness.

Detailed below are four quite different approaches which all claim considerable success. None of these treatments is recognised by trichologists in Britain but they have proved successful in clinical trials, and some are used by dermatologists or are common treatments abroad.

NOURKRIN

As a newcomer to Britain, Nourkrin has yet to make its mark. The product which has enjoyed remarkable success in its native Finland has been available here for less than a year – not long enough to prove its efficacy. Nourkrin is basically a food supplement, not a drug. It contains fish cartilage (which contains **polysaccharides** – the reduction of these chemicals has been linked to thinning hair), other marine extracts, silica, vitamin C and trace elements. It was developed in Finland by Professor Alan Lassus, a dermatologist at Helsinki University, and has been available in Finland and Norway since 1992 under the brand name of Viviscal. Since then Professor Lassus claims it has been phenomenally successful and is now recommended by traditionally conservative Scandinavian dermatologists instead of minoxidil which, he claims, 'just doesn't sell any more'.

Controlled double-blind clinical tests in Finland revealed favourable results. The tests were carried out on forty men, average age twenty-five, all with male pattern baldness. Half of the men were given two tablets of Nourkrin every day for six months; the other half were given a harmless fish extract tablet. The results, published in the *International Journal of Medical Research*, showed that the men on Nourkrin reported an average hair increase of 38 percent while the men taking the fish extract reported only 2 percent. Similar tests on older men also showed successful hair growth but the growth was slower. Smokers didn't do very well, which is not surprising as smoking is a vasoconstrictor (it causes blood vessels to contract, which prevents the hair from getting the nutrients it needs). Nourkrin is still undergoing trials in Belgium, Sweden and at Yale University, but so far no clinical trials have been conducted in Britain. Although there are no known side-effects to Nourkrin, some people may not be able to take it if they are allergic to fish.

Success is dosage-dependent. It takes an average of two tablets a day to produce results, although people who smoke or are larger or older than average may need to take more. It also takes a minimum of three months to notice any improvements and you'll need to keep taking the tablets indefinitely to maintain that improvement.

Nourkrin is available from Selfridges, large pharmacies or direct from the distributors Pharma Health and Beauty UK (see Useful Addresses).

NATURAL HAIR PRODUCTS

The Natural Hair Products (NHP) programme seems complicated in theory but users testify to its simplicity in practice.

Unlike the Nourkrin, minoxidil or surgical treatments, the approach of NHP is very much a way of life rather than a quick-fix approach and as such it appeals to dedicated hair growers only.

The theory

NHP is the brain child of Andy Bryant who became a minor celebrity in 1994 when he had a vasectomy under hypnosis. Andy, who had been losing his own hair for a few years, was unconvinced by the orthodox explanation of the reasons for male pattern baldness and the acceptable approach to treatment. He spent five years of serious research into the subject and came up with what he believes are the causes of hair loss: poor blood supply, muscular tension, poor nutrition, sluggish lymphatic system and stress.

The main determinant in all of these is stress, or rather our response to stress. 'Baldness is not a separate condition but an external sign of the body as a whole.' It is true, he argues, that hormones have an effect, but the effect is on the entire body not just on the hair follicle. Increased testosterone released from puberty onwards acts on the brain and the moods, causing increased levels of aggression and competitiveness. A man's mood affects how he reacts to stress and feeling tense brings about a high stress level and causes vasoconstriction which ultimately results in hair loss. Women's lower testosterone levels are counteracted by oestrogen until after the menopause. But women under extreme stress can also grow more body hair while the hair on their heads gets thinner.

The practice

The NHP programme follows a system known as SIDES which stands for Stress, Inversion, Diet, Exercise and Shampoo.

Stress, or rather how you handle it, affects the quality of your hair because it causes vasoconstriction. To combat its ill-effects NHP recommends exercise, relaxation techniques, sleep and a five-year life plan, whereby you set goals for your relationships, work, finances, etc. NHP also provides stress monitors – little plastic devices that you stick on the inside of your arm – to register your levels of stress.

Inversion is simply hanging upside down for a matter of seconds every day to enable blood to flow more easily to and from the scalp, so that nutrients get to the scalp and waste products drain away. You can do this by either bending forwards so that your head hangs upside down or by using an inverter – a tilting table which is sold by NHP. Whatever form of inversion you choose it's important to feel secure and stress-free. NHP claims that its inverter is finely tuned to allow the right amount of vasodilation, but trichologists disagree. Some say that inversion has a temporary effect only and the inverter is an expensive and useless piece of machinery. The inverter costs from £335, which makes it the most expensive part of the £423 (inc VAT) programme.

Diet should be high in water, rich in vital hair nutrients and low in artificial stimulants such as coffee and alcohol. Top of the diet sheet come fruit, vegetables, salad and at least eight glasses of water a day. The programme recommends eating a good diet and avoiding vitamin crazes.

Exercise includes scalp exercises to encourage blood flow and reduce scalp tension. It also includes introducing more exercise into your life to reduce tension and boost blood flow.

Shampoo should be as close as possible to the natural pH of the scalp, which is between 5.0 and 5.6.

Replace the inverter with gentle massage and the advice given by NHP is basically the same advice many top trichologists give for keeping your hair healthy. The difference is that trichologists don't believe following this type of diet and lifestyle programme can reverse the effects of genetic hair loss. NHP has no clinical studies to back up its claims, but there are around 950 people following the programme at the moment. It can take up to nine months to notice any improvement. Men and women who have been following the programme for two years say their hair and their health has improved enormously. Less stress, better skin, loss of weight, better sleep and fewer minor illnesses are just some of the benefits they claim. For more information contact Natural Health Products Ltd (see Useful Addresses).

PHYTOLOGIE

Phytologie is a range of plant-based products from France. Again, it is a relative newcomer to Britain. The range contains two hair loss products that claim to treat the problem rather than cure it: Phytocyane and Phytopolléïne Plus. Of these, Phytopolléïne Plus is the more potent. Phytocyane is aimed at women and is really for acute hair loss while Phytopolléïne Plus is a concentrated formula for chronic hair loss.

Phytopolléïne Plus contains a blend of eight plant essential oils chosen for their antiseptic, healing, anti-inflammatory and vasculotonic (boosts the vascular system) properties, trace elements, amino acids and plant placenta extract. The result of ten years' research by dermatologists, chemical engineers and pharmacists, was originally used by dermatologists. It is now used by the Institute of Trichologists in France and is endorsed by the French Ministry of Health.

The theory behind Phytopolléïne Plus is that it enables you to keep your hair for longer by strengthening existing hair to extend the anagen (growth) phase of the hair. You will still go bald eventually if you have been genetically programmed to do so, but it will take much longer, maybe ten or twenty years longer. Phytopolléïne Plus works by improving the health of the scalp, stimulating the hair bulb and regulating the amount of sebum produced. The product is totally natural and there are no side-effects.

Three series of clinical trials conducted on both men and women at the St Louis Hospital in Paris and the Hospital of Montmorency showed favourable results for Phytopolléïne Plus. The third, and most recent, series used the most sophisticated testing techniques. It was carried out in 1986 on thirty-two men with male pattern baldness between stages two and five (see Chapter 2) and reinforced the findings of the two previous trials.

In each of these trials the product was applied twice a week, the night before shampooing, for six months. The results were positive, and when taken together with the previous two tests showed that, overall, women responded better than men and young men responded better than older men. Seventy-nine percent of women showed some improvement compared with 63 percent of men. When the results were broken down into three distinct areas of improvement: 24 percent of men had stopped losing hair and were showing some signs of regrowth after the six-month period, 27 percent were losing noticeably less hair than before the trial and 12 percent were losing moderately less hair than before.

Phytopolléïne Plus is available from selected stockists (see Phyto Distribution UK under Useful Addresses). You need to take Phytopolléïne Plus for at least three months before you notice any improvement. The Phytologie range also includes Phytophanére, a dietary supplement that includes a combination of vitamins, essential fatty acids, amino acids and minerals. Phytologie also favours the general advice to reduce stress, improve your diet and follow sensible hair-care guidelines.

KEVIS

Kevis Lotion is part of a hair-care package that includes shampoo and two sets of powdered vitamin and mineral supplements – one is a vitamin boost for hair, the other is an anti-stress formulation.

It is the lotion that has attracted most attention. It includes amino acids to hydrate the scalp and hair; sulphur, which is essential for making keratin; biotin and sodium pantothenate, which are important for cell metabolism, a naturally occurring vasodilator and other ingredients to restore the levels of mucopolysaccharides on the scalp to the anagen growth phase. It is marketed as a lotion for thinning hair but has also shown positive results in clinical trials on men and women experiencing male pattern baldness.

Over thirty clinical trials have been carried out on Kevis Lotion; the following one was carried out and involved 100 men aged between eighteen and fifty, all of whom were receding at the hairline and had begun to thin at the crown.

The group was divided into two groups of fifty. One group was treated with Kevis, one with a placebo. All the participants in the Kevis group massaged one ampoule of Kevis into the bald and surrounding areas once a day for three months, while the placebo group did the same with another, harmless liquid.

After three months, various tests confirmed that Kevis had reduced hair fall and strengthened the existing hair. The period was too short to assess significant levels of regrowth but 70 percent of the Kevis trialists said they were satisfied or very satisfied with the results, compared with 31 percent of the placebo group.

For information on Kevis, contact Romanda Healthcare (see Useful Addresses).

Note on Clinical Trials

It is a complicated procedure to try to evaluate such a dynamic phenomenon as hair growth. And over the years many methods have been tried, tested and subsequently discredited. The current accepted form of measuring hair growth in clinical trials is by using a phototrichogram.

This photographic technique enables the tester to take a close-up photograph of a defined area of the scalp (about $1cm^2$ or $2cm^2$) where the hairs have been cut or shaved off. The hairs in the area are photographed and counted before, during and after treatment to assess the efficacy of a treatment. The technique also enables the tester to determine the length of the hair growth cycles. The products in this chapter that have undergone clinical trials have been assessed in this way, but not all the products on the market have.

Ultimately, no matter what the tests prove, if you do not grow back visible, strong, healthy hair then the product hasn't worked.

Finding Your Way Round the Small Ads

Newspapers and magazines are littered with advertisements for products that claim to grow your hair back. Some of these can help to prolong the life of your hair, but many cannot.

Advertising is a legitimate and closely regulated form of selling. Advertisements for drugs and vitamins must be passed by either the Pharmaceutical Association of Great Britain (PAGB) or the Medicines Control Agency (MCA), although creams and lotions are more difficult to regulate. Therefore responsible companies will make only legitimate claims for their products. But if you want to play safe don't buy products that make miraculous claims – your hair is not going to grow back in six weeks when healthy hair grows only half an inch in a month – better still, take the advice of a professional, either a trichologist, dermatologist or registered alternative practitioner.

─── 5 ───

How to Keep Your Hair

Apart from the skilled surgery, drugs and the many alternative techniques that aim to help you defeat hair loss there are simple steps that everyone can take to slow down the hairloss process. It doesn't take much skill or cost a lot of money, it simply requires giving a little thought to what you eat, how you live and how much care you actually take of your hair.

A healthy body will be low in cholesterol and boast excellent blood circulation. Circulation is important as blood carries nutrients all around the body, and to the roots of the hair – a healthy hair is a well-nourished hair. Together with the lymphatic system the blood also carries away waste products to be excreted. What we eat has a direct effect on how efficiently the circulatory system works.

Exercise also boosts both circulation and the lymphatic system, which is the body's drainage system. And when it comes to personal grooming, let's face it, most of us either neglect our hair or batter it into submission. We stretch it, scorch it, twist it, perm it, colour it and brush it, all in the name of fashion, and yet we ignore its poor condition, scaly scalp and falling hairs until it's too late. If you really want to keep your hair, give it some of the attention it deserves.

Diet

Because of the low status of hair in the body's hierarchy, the goodness in your diet will go to support the more vital body functions before it reaches your hair. So it follows that the better your diet the better the condition and quantity of your hair. And, although male pattern baldness is an exception to this rule, improvements in diet and lifestyle can delay or slow down hair loss in some people.

It is not just a matter of eating the right foods, it is also important to eat good quality food. Organic produce is slightly more expensive than the mass-produced variety and doesn't look as squeaky clean but eating organic means you are less likely to ingest a battery of hazardous chemicals. Food is fuel for the body, which is more amazing than the most sophisticated piece of machinery ever designed. So just as you wouldn't expect your high-performance Ferrari to run on low-grade petrol, you can't feed your body rubbish and expect it to be in peak condition.

The general rules are to avoid products containing saturated fats, refined sugars, white flour and caffeine and not to eat too many overprocessed foods or animal products. Aim for a balanced diet of wholegrain breads, cereals, brown rice and pasta. Eat at least five daily helpings of fresh fruit and vegetables, packed with vitamins (including the vital **antioxidants**), and drink plenty of water. In addition, try to eat fish once or twice a week, preferably oily fish such as mackerel, tuna or sardines, which are high in essential fatty acids. Among other things they lower blood cholesterol, improve circulation and have an anti-inflammatory effect which is beneficial for dry scalp conditions such as dermatitis (dandruff). This type of diet has been shown to protect against disease, and the nutrients recommended for good health are also important for good hair.

Vitamins for Hair

In addition to a good basic diet, there are many vitamins, minerals and amino acids which have been singled out as essential for good hair. These all have different roles to play: some are beneficial for the scalp, others fight the battle against grey hair and many more improve the integrity of hair generally, boosting the condition, shine, body and thickness. Yet more are beneficial for hair loss, but it depends very much on the reason for the loss. As with any other form of treatment you need to know the reason for your hair loss before you can begin to address it. That's why it is usually best to consult a nutritional therapist who can assess your individual needs. He or she will work out a programme of nutrition for you, which takes into account the state of your health, your nutritional deficiencies and your ability to absorb certain vitamins.

It is of course possible to take a range of vitamin and mineral supplements at home, and thousands of people do. But there are two main flaws in self-prescribing. One is that you could take a variety of recommended vitamin and mineral supplements and still lack the basic ingredient that is vital to your nutritional needs. The other is that certain supplements can cancel each other out so that you either get no benefits or a very poor balance.

So, if you do take vitamin pills, play safe and take as few as possible.

The vitamins, minerals, amino acids and herbs listed below are recognised as important in preventing hair loss generally. This list is intended as a guide only and is no substitute for professional advice. The new, updated recommended daily allowances (RDAs) are given where appropriate, but many nutritional therapists and health practitioners consider them still to be too low. RDAs are set at a level to stave off deficiency-related diseases, they are not targets for optimum health. You can safely boost your levels by eating an extra portion of vegetables, a small mixed salad, a couple of pieces of fruit and a glass of fruit juice every day. But if you plan to alter your diet radically or splash out on a vast range of nutritional supplements you should consult a nutritional therapist. You can find a nutritional therapist through the Society for the Promotion of Nutritional Therapy (see Useful Addresses).

Vitamin B complex (includes niacin, biotin, inositol, choline and pantothenic acid). All of the B vitamins are important for healthy hair. Lack of any of them can result in a scaly scalp, thin hair and hair loss. But even among the B complex vitamins, certain specific vitamins have been singled out as being particularly beneficial to hair. **Biotin** is so popular as an anti-baldness vitamin that it has been isolated and used in hair products for topical application. Biotin slows down hair loss, boosts hair growth, helps hormone production, helps synthesise fatty acids and boosts metabolism. Biotin deficiency is rare, but where it occurs it can lead to seborrhoeic dermatitis. **Niacin – vitamin B3** – with hawthorn berry can stimulate the vascular system, boost circulation and can be of value in age-related hair loss. **Inositol** is essential for hair growth and also prevents hair loss. It also regulates cholesterol and helps to metabolise fats, all of which boost circulation. It is not a 'true' vitamin because it can be made in the body. It is found in abundance in male reproductive organs, particularly in semen. **Choline** is not a 'true B' either. It helps with the accumulation of sebum which can get impacted in the follicles and helps to facilitate the removal of accumulated fats from the liver. **Pantothenic acid – vitamin B5** – is good for stress-induced hair loss and also helps to prevent dermatitis.

Good food sources: **biotin** – liver, milk, cheese, eggs, brewer's yeast, and yeast extract. RDA 0.15mg, but you may need more if you're under great stress or taking antibiotics. **Niacin** – cheese, milk, yeast extract, fortified breakfast cereals and brewer's yeast. RDA 18mg; heavy drinkers may need more. **Inositol** – liver, steak, brewer's yeast, citrus fruits, nuts and pulses. There is no RDA and it is very difficult to overdose. **Choline** is found in the same foods and likewise there is no RDA. **Pantothenic acid** – brewer's yeast, brown rice, pulses and eggs. RDA 6mg.

Cautions: The B vitamins tend to work as a team, so it's important to maintain a balance as too much of one can result in too little of another. They all tend to be found in similar foods, although in differing quantities. If in doubt go for fish, offal, wholegrains and yeast extract. If you need to supplement your diet, choose a good B-complex supplement and ask for nutritional guidance, if necessary.

Zinc is a trace element necessary for absorbing other vitamins, especially vitamins A and the B complex, and to help enzymes to work. It is also important for growth and helps the development of sex organs. Lack of zinc can result in hair loss.

Good food sources: oysters and other seafood, liver, meat and dairy products, bee pollen, garlic and seeds. The RDA is 15mg, which one portion of liver, chicken or seafood will provide.

Iodine plays a major role in regulating the thyroid gland; imbalances in thyroid function can cause hair loss. It also helps to determine the rate at which our body works. Lack of iodine can lead to a sluggish metabolism and hair loss.

Good food sources: seaweed, seafood and fish oils. RDA 150mcg.

Cysteine is an amino acid that makes up about 8 percent of hair. It works in a combination of ways; it breaks down fatty acids and also strengthens the hair.

Good food sources: Eggs are the best natural source. You can also get it in beans, meat and legumes. But people with really weak hair will need to take supplements of between 500 and 1,000mg.

Silica is also very effective, especially when combined with cysteine. Silica is found in the hair cuticle and is also present in human skin. It has been shown to be a component of **mucopolysaccharides**, starches which occur in higher levels in young skin and young, thick hair.

Good sources: You will probably have to take supplements of organic silica as it is not something we can get from food. We only need small amounts of this important mineral, which is the most prevalent element on earth after oxygen. There is no RDA, but in a clinical trial conducted to assess the importance of silica in ageing skin, fragile hair and brittle nails, good results were achieved with a daily dose of 10ml of a liquid silica supplement called Silicol. Other silica and silicon supplements are available in tablet form.

Iron improves your resistance to stress and boosts circulation. Lack of iron caused by heavy periods can cause hair loss and trichologists have always known that true anaemia can cause hair loss.

Good food sources: liver, spinach, sardines, fortified breakfast cereals, dried apricots. Vitamin C helps the body to absorb iron, so drinking a glass of orange juice with your meals can help you get the most from your food. RDA 14mg, which is obtainable from 350g of dried apricots or boiled spinach.

Psoralea is a Chinese herb which boosts hair growth. It is available as a herb from Chinese herbalists, but is not available as a supplement. Clinical trials using extract of psoralea for male pattern baldness are in progress, so it may one day be used as a treatment.

Saw palmetto is a herb that is believed to inhibit the conversion of testosterone into dihydrotestosterone. So far there have been no clinical trials in relation to hair loss, but clinical trials using saw palmetto as a treatment for enlarged prostate have had favourable results – dihydrotestosterone, which is responsible for the onset of male pattern baldness, is also the hormone that causes enlarged prostate. Quite high doses would be required to delay hair loss and it may also be possible to apply the herb topically to the scalp, although it is a highly coloured berry that may cause staining. If you want to try saw palmetto, it is best to consult a registered herbalist – contact the National Institute of Medical Herbalists (see Useful Addresses).

Antioxidants

The antioxidant vitamins A (in the form of beta-carotene), vitamins C and E and the minerals selenium and zinc, found in green, red and yellow fruit and vegetables, are widely recognised as some of our greatest allies in the fight against disease. But they are also recognised as the great protectors against ageing and its related effects such as wrinkling and hair loss. American age researchers Durk Pearson and Sandy Shaw have been using massive doses of antioxidants to treat male pattern baldness and other hair disorders. The results have been encouraging.

Pearson and Shaw are also famous for their use of Polysorbate 80, an emulsifier used in mayonnaise. They discovered that Polysorbate 80 blended with vitamins biotin and niacin and applied to balding areas of the scalp caused a histamine release, which is necessary for cell growth. They claim hundreds of men used the mixture daily and over 60 percent of them noticed regrowth within three months. Pearson and Shaw's methods are generally not recognised by trichologists. Their tests have proved, however, that certain vitamins, minerals and amino acids are critical to healthy hair. They discuss antioxidants and Polysorbate 80 in detail in their best-selling book *Life Extension* (Warner Books).

A Note on Protein

You may have heard that protein is vital for good hair. Of course it is, but its importance is often overestimated. A shortage of protein can cause hair to deteriorate and even fall out, but very few people in the developed world are likely to run short of protein. In fact, most people consume far more protein than their body needs. A cooked breakfast of bacon, eggs and toast and a cup of tea with milk provides enough protein for the day. Eating too much protein puts extra stress on the body as it has to be broken down and its toxic waste excreted.

Water

Our bodies are 50–75 percent water and we should aim to drink at least eight glasses of water a day to keep this level topped up and to help flush waste products from the body. If that sounds too unappealing you can have the occasional glass of sparkling or flavoured mineral water or mix it with fruit juice. But try to avoid tea, coffee, caffeine-laden fizzy drinks and alcohol. These are all diuretics – they dehydrate rather than moisturise the body.

Water is a vital but often forgotten nutrient in good health and is as important to healthy hair as it is to plump, well-moisturised skin. It is also the major component of perspiration. When we exercise we perspire and this stimulates the sebaceous glands of the hair follicles to produce oil which moisturises the hair shaft.

Stress

As we saw in Chapter 2 stress affects every area of our life and health and can cause hair loss in people of all ages, or cause increased loss in people who are already losing hair through illness, childbirth or male pattern baldness. It is true for example that many men will lose their hair eventually because they are genetically programmed to do so, but excess stress can elevate androgens in the system so they might lose it sooner, at twenty rather than thirty or at thirty rather than forty. So, although it is difficult to claim that reducing stress levels can prevent baldness, it can help you to hold on to what you've got for longer.

It is natural to feel anxious when you find you are losing your hair, but anxiety will only add to the problem, so the first step is not to panic. The second step is to identify the areas of stress in your life. Make a list of all the aspects of your life that worry you, put them in order of which worries you most and ask yourself what you can do about them. It is not always possible or even desirable to remove the cause of your stress as it might be your job or an important relationship, but you can change how you handle it, and you must learn to relax so you don't stay in a permanent state of anxiety.

Visualisation, yoga, meditation and exercise can all help you to relax, reducing the destructive effects of stress on your body, while time management, planning, prioritising and delegating can help you work more efficiently so you have less to worry about. You can't do everything, so do what's most important and leave the rest to someone else and accept that there are some things you just can't change.

Remember also that you are not alone. Stress is an epidemic in this country, so there are stress management, yoga and meditation classes nationwide. Ask at your local library for details of classes or speak to your GP. Many fund-holding GPs are referring patients to yoga and meditation classes as a safer and healthier alternative to drugs. A full body aromatherapy massage is a wonderful indulgence with a fabulous feel-good factor. A professional therapist will use oils with specific relaxation properties to bring about a deep sense of well-being. At home you can use six or seven drops of lavender, camomile or geranium essential oils in your bath to help you wind down after a stressful day.

Head Massage

Massaging the scalp boosts circulation and encourages fresh blood supplies to flow to the surface of the scalp and feed the hair follicles. It also reduces tension. Oil is not necessary unless you are completely bald or want to use a stimulating tonic such as one of those mentioned below. Massaging once a week has a beneficial effect on your hair and also helps you to relax.

This massage is based on one from leading trichologist Philip Kingsley. It is quick and easy so you can do it yourself or, even better, ask someone to do it for you. Use it when your scalp feels tense, when you feel under stress generally or simply when you wash your hair.

* Place the pads of your fingertips, not your nails, firmly on your scalp at the front of your hair line and spread your fingers.

* Keeping your hands in one place, move your fingers in a spreading and contracting action, as if you were kneading dough, firmly but gently, without scratching or irritating the scalp. Massage that area for about a minute.

* Using this kneading technique, work your way through the scalp over the forehead and above the ears, then over the crown and down to the nape of the neck, spending about a minute on each area. This follows the direction of the blood flow to the heart.

* Finish at the back of the neck. Your scalp should feel tingly and relaxed.

Hair Tonics

Hair tonics have been used for generations to improve the condition and appearance of the hair. Using a tonic in conjunction with a weekly massage can boost its effects as well as provide specific benefits to the hair. Indian head masseurs have been using massage combined with herbal lotions for over 1,000 years to relieve tension in the scalp and neck and promote thick, healthy hair. Indian herbal oils are also available in this country. Narendra Mehta, the man who brought Indian head massage to Britain, recommends Shalocks Ayurvedic Precious Herbal Hair Oil, which contains a combination of Indian herbs to prevent dandruff, promote a healthy scalp and boost hair growth. The lotion is available from Harrods.

You could also make up your own lotion from essential oils. Robert Tisserand recommends the following aromatherapy lotion once or twice a week for six to eight weeks: seven drops of juniper oil, five drops of lemon grass, five drops of eucalyptus and twelve drops of rosemary diluted in 30ml of a vegetable carrier oil of your choice (such as almond or grapeseed). Rub it into the scalp and massage gently with your finger tips for three to four minutes. Leave in for at least half an hour, or overnight, if you wish, then shampoo off. The lotion will leave your hair very greasy so when you come to wash it massage a small amount of shampoo into your hair and scalp before you wet your hair. This emulsifies the oils, making them easier to remove.

All the oils in this lotion are natural stimulants which boost circulation in the scalp and encourage growth in lazy hair roots. This is an effective lotion but like most forms of treatment it doesn't work for everyone. If you have noticed no improvement after six weeks of use, then it isn't going to work, so there is no point in using it again. Those who do find it helpful should use it in blocks of six to eight weeks two or three times a year, but don't keep using it indefinitely.

Choosing and Using the Right Shampoo

If you have read much other information on hair care you will probably have come across the advice not to use a detergent-based shampoo. This will be difficult to achieve as all shampoos are, in fact, detergents. A detergent is simply anything that will remove oil and dirt and if it doesn't it's not doing its job. Shampoos, shower gels, soap, washing-up liquid and washing powder are all detergents with various degrees of stripping and cleaning ability. The difference lies in the type of detergent used and the harshness of the product.

Detergent-based shampoo became a household product at the turn of the century thanks to the dedication of Massachusetts fireman John Breck, a man with a mission to nip his own baldness in the bud. Needless to say he went on to develop other hair and scalp products which were a huge success. Before Breck most people used soap, which wasn't very successful as it left behind a rather nasty scum.

Today, there is a huge gulf between the best and worst shampoos: some are almost akin to washing-up liquid while others are so sophisticated you can use them as often as you like. Shampoos are simply a combination of **surfactants**, which are the cleansers, and a variable amount of extras to give smell, colour and conditioning ability. A good shampoo will clean your hair with the minimum of damage.

Often the advice to use a non-detergent-based shampoo means to use a shampoo made from natural products.

Unfortunately, we have come to expect a frenzy of foam from our shampoos. Foam is characteristic of shampoos that use petrochemical surfactants which strip the hair of its protective sebaceous coating. But there are many other shampoos that use natural detergents such as sodium laureth sulphate, derived from coconut oil. This is a natural and effective cleanser used by many companies which make plant- and aromatherapy-based products.

Hair-thickening Products

Hair-thickening shampoos may temporarily make hair look thicker. They usually contain protein, and some which contain panthenol, or pro-vitamin B5, can increase the diameter of the hair shaft by up to 10 percent. Panthenol, which is present in the living cells of plants and animals, attracts moisture to the hair. Trichologists have mixed feelings about hair-thickening products.

Some would say that shampoo is a poor vehicle for thickening ingredients because you put it on, rinse it off and very little clings to the hair. Others believe that these products can benefit as the hair will swell by up to 30 percent when it is wet and a shampoo that contains thickening additives can both cling on to and penetrate the wet hair shaft.

Thickening lotions can have more of a cosmetic effect because the thickening ingredients have more time to act.

Spray-on hair thickeners which come in an assortment of colours have the effect of making the hair look slightly fuller and they also colour the scalp beneath to give the appearance of a full head of hair. The result is purely cosmetic and not very effective at that. Hair thickeners do not make your hair grow better or thicker and have no lasting value.

TEN STEPS TO CLEAN AND HEALTHY HAIR

1   Use a gentle plant-based shampoo when possible or a very small amount of a good quality petrochemical alternative. Don't expect a lot of foam – foam is no indication of effective cleansing. Don't be swayed by labels that claim to be for frequent use, the surfactants used can be as harsh or as gentle as those used in any other type of shampoo.

2   Choose a product that suits your hair type. If you have a problem with dandruff you can control it with a coal tar shampoo. The latest shampoos containing tea tree essential oil also have a natural cleansing and antiseptic effect on the scalp, as does an infusion of nettle and the herb rosemary. Another delicious natural alternative is to add eight drops of rose geranium oil, eight drops of lemon oil and eight drops of rosemary oil to a 250ml bottle of the purest, unperfumed shampoo you can find and use that.

3   The amount of shampoo you use depends on the length of your hair and the number of styling products you need to wash out of it, but most people use too much shampoo. Use only a small amount (about the size of a ten-pence piece) in the palm of your hand and rub well into thoroughly wet hair, massaging but not scrubbing your scalp as you wash. Rinse your hair thoroughly until it squeaks and towel dry very gently to avoid pulling or wringing the hair.

TEN STEPS TO CLEAN AND HEALTHY HAIR

4   How often you should wash your hair is a matter of hot debate. Some trichologists say the new mild shampoos mean you can wash your hair three times a day if you want, especially since the massaging action and possibly the act of bending over the bath or sink encourages the flow of nutrients to the follicle, but others disagree, saying that you can in fact overstimulate the scalp and weaken the hair. Fabienne Osswald, a leading French hair specialist, recommends washing only once a week. She believes washing your hair every day not only subjects it to the detergents and chemicals in the shampoo, but also to the pollution in the water and possibly the daily trauma of heated styling products. You might be best advised to moderate between these two extremes. If you shampoo every day, try it every other day instead to see if your hair improves in quality and appearance.

5   Use a conditioner and rinse it out well. Conditioner won't mend broken hair, but it does smooth the hair shaft making it easier to comb and less susceptible to damage. Conditioner is essential for dry hair.

TEN STEPS TO CLEAN AND HEALTHY HAIR

6	Comb, don't brush your hair when it is wet. Brushing stretches wet hair and can cause breakages. It is best to comb with a wide-tooth saw-cut comb, where each tooth is cut into the comb leaving no sharp or rough edges. Most saw-cut combs are made of plastic, but it's better to use those made from hard rubber (vulcanite). The best combs are made from horn, ivory or tortoiseshell. But these are very expensive and not very animal or environmentally friendly.
7	Using a very soft, natural bristle brush, turn your head upside down and brush through very gently at night. This will gently detangle the hair, remove loose particles of dust, and encourage blood flow to the scalp while you brush the stronger hair underneath.
8	Massage your scalp daily or weekly as indicated above.
9	Eat a diet that encourages healthy hair and get nutritional advice if you think you need it.
10	Take regular, cardiovascular exercise to boost circulation and work off stress. Exercise is one of the many non-specific ways of improving your hair. Remember, if it is good for your health, it is good for your hair.

Wigs – Cover-Ups or Confidence Boosters?

If you are bald and feel very self-conscious about it, a wig can help to boost confidence, but apart from that they are generally not a good idea. Wigs have had a notoriously bad name. The outrageous creations of the eighteenth-century Court of Versailles in France were so big and heavy that mice nested in them and they sometimes caused fatal abscesses where they rested on the temples. Even in more recent years they are often ill-fitting, badly designed, poor-quality synthetic creations. But you can get good-quality wigs, at a price. Those that look and feel best are made from real hair. Unfortunately, they are also very expensive and take some looking after but you don't get that woolly hat feel that you can get with synthetic wigs.

Wig wearers can suffer from irritation and itchiness of the scalp. If you do wear a wig take it off whenever you can, wash your scalp every night as wigs make your head sweat, and keep your wig clean, especially the underside. Real hair wigs need to be kept on a wig block to keep their shape and they should be shampooed and conditioned every two weeks.

Prices for real hair wigs vary but you can expect to pay at least £400. People who need wigs for medical reasons can get them on the National Health Service at substantially reduced prices, and they are free to people on income support.

For a list of registered wig fitters and suppliers contact the Liaison Officer at HMWA (see Useful Addresses).

Glossary

Alopecia Hair loss.

Alopecia areata Round patches of hair loss on the scalp, beard or eyebrows which get bigger as the condition develops.

Amino acid Basic units in the structure of proteins. Of the twenty common amino acids, eight cannot be made by the body, so they must come from food. These are called essential amino acids.

Anagen The growth phase in the hair cycle.

Antioxidant A compound that protects tissue from destructive rogue molecules called free radicals. Vitamins A, C, E and trace elements zinc and selenium are antioxidants.

Auto-immune disease Disease where the body's immune system breaks down and destroys its own cells, eg rheumatoid arthritis.

Catagen The rest phase in the hair cycle that precedes hair fall.

Diffuse alopecia Hair is lost from all over the scalp area in a sort of thinning-out process as opposed to bald patches.

Dihydrotestosterone Another name for androgen, the hormone that influences hair loss.

5 alpha reductase The enzyme that acts on testosterone to change it into androgen.

Follicle A pit-like structure in the skin which contains the living part of the hair and which is linked to the sebaceous gland.

Holistic treatment Any form of treatment that treats the whole person – mind, body, spirit and lifestyle – rather than just the symptoms.

Keratin A fibrous proetin that forms the body's horny tissues, such as fingernails. Keratin is also found in hair.

Lanugo Fine colourless hair that covers the foetus in the womb.

Lymphatic system A system of small vessels that travel around the body giving nourishment and taking away waste.

Papillae Clumps of cells which produce the hair cells that keratinise, die and form the hair shaft.

Polysaccharides and mucopolysaccharides Groups of carbohydrates which make up part of the hair shaft believed to be important in the growth phase of hair.

Sebaceous gland The gland linked to the hair follicle which secretes sebum on the shaft of the hair and on the scalp.

Sebum The oil secreted by the sebaceous gland which moisturises the skin and hair.

Surfactant A substance that acts on the surface of the hair and scalp to remove dirt and oil.

Telogen The phase in the hair cycle when it is normal for hair to fall out.

Terminal hair The coarse, coloured protective hair that grows on the scalp. Eyebrows, eyelashes, pubic hair and beards are also terminal hair.

Traction alopecia Hair loss as a result of the hair being pulled out by the root, often caused by styling.

Trichologist A hair and scalp specialist.

Vasoconstrictor Something that causes the blood vessels to contract so that the passage of blood and the oxygen and nutrients carried in it are restricted. Stress and smoking are vasoconstrictors.

Vasodilator Something, such as relaxation and certain nutrients, which causes the blood vessels to expand and so boosts circulation.

Vellus hair The first hair that grows after birth. It is fine, soft and colourless and rarely more than 2cm long. It covers all the body apart from the palms of the hands, soles of the feet and lips.

Useful Addresses

The British Complementary Medicine Association
Exmoor Street
London W10 6DZ
Tel: 0181 964 1205

Hairline International
The Alopecia Patients Support Group
Lyons Court
1668 High Street
Knole
West Midlands BN3 0LY
(send a SAE for information)
Alopecia helpline: 01564 775 281

HMWA, Wig Makers' Section
6 Gales Close
Merrow Park
Guildford
Surrey GU4 7EG

Institute for Complementary Medicine
PO Box 194
London SE16 1QZ
(send an SAE and three loose first-class stamps for information)
Tel: 0171 237 5165

The Institute of Trichologists
228 Stockwell Road
London SW9 9SU
(include an SAE for details)
Tel: 0171 733 2056

National Institute of Medical Herbalists
Dept H
9 Palace Gate
Exeter EX1 1JA
Tel: 01392 426 022

Natural Hair Products Ltd
The Hook
Cedar Road
Woking
Surrey GU22 0JJ
Tel: 01483 725702
Helpline: 0891 505 118

Pharma Health and Beauty UK Ltd (for Nourkrin)
PO Box 3379
London SW11 3ED
Tel: 0171 223 1665

Phyto Distribution UK (for Phytologie)
15 Cleveland Square
London W2 6DG
Tel: 0171 402 0717 for your nearest Phytologie stockist

Romanda Healthcare (for Kevis Lotion)
Romanda House
Ashley Walk
London NW7 1DU
Advice line: 0181 346 0784

Dr Hugh Rushton, FIT
22 Harley Street
London W1N 1AP
Tel: 0171 637 0491

Society for the Promotion of Nutritional Therapy
First Floor
The Enterprise Centre
Station Parade
Eastbourne BN21 1BE
Tel: 01323 430 203

The Trichological Centre
28–32 Princess Street
Manchester M1 4LB
Tel: 0161 228 0657

Index